FROM MED STUDENT TO MEDICAL MARVEL

Habits of Highly Effective Learners

COPYRIGHT

2024 SOLV MKT All rights reserved.

No part of this publication may be reproduced, distributed, or transmitted in any form or by any means, including photocopying, recording, or other electronic or mechanical methods, without the prior written permission of the publisher, except in the case of brief quotations embodied in reviews and certain other non-commercial uses permitted by copyright law.

CATALOG

- COPYRIGHT 2
- **Part 1** 4
- **How a Medical Marvel Thinks** 4
  - Chapter 1 5
  - Embracing the Medical Journey 5
  - From Goal to Reality 5
  - Chapter 2 9
  - How to Develop a Growth Mindset and Love Challenges 9
  - Chapter 3 12
  - Unleashing Your Drive 12
  - How to Learn for the Rest of Your Life 12
- **Part 2** 17
- **How to Get Good at Medical Knowledge** 17
  - Chapter 4 18
  - Mastering Time Management 18
  - Taking on the Coursework 18
  - Chapter 5 25
  - Strategies for Active Learning 25
  - Getting Involved with the Material 25
  - Chapter 6 31
  - Getting More Knowledge 31
  - Textbooks, Lectures, and More 31
- **Part 3** 38
- **Improving What You Remember and Can Remember** 38
  - Chapter 7 39
  - The Power of Practice: More Than Just Reading 39
  - Chapter 8 44
  - Memory Magic 44
  - How to Remember Things for a Long Time 44
  - Chapter 9 51
  - Working Together To Learn 51
  - Teaching and Learning With Other People 51
- **Part 4** 57
- **Habits for Well-Rounded Success Outside of School** 57
  - Chapter 10 58
  - Taking Care of Yourself: Keeping Your Mind and Body Healthy ... 58
  - Chapter 11 64
  - Putting together Strong Support Systems 64
  - Family, Friends, and Mentors 64
  - Chapter 12 70
  - Finding Balance 70
  - A Life Outside of Medicine 70
- **General Tips for Readers** 76

Part 1

How a Medical Marvel Thinks

CHAPTER 1
EMBRACING THE MEDICAL JOURNEY
From Goal to Reality

Thanks for taking the plunge into this exciting journey! You've made it to medical school, the first step toward your goal of becoming a doctor. You will learn the things, gain the skills, and feel the kindness you need to heal others and have a huge effect on many lives on this journey.

This chapter will help you get started with your medical education by giving you a road plan. We'll talk about what to expect, focus on key skills for success, and get you excited about the amazing road that lies ahead.

From Hope to Commitment

To become a doctor, you need a spark of motivation, like a desire to help people in pain, an interest in the human body, or a desire to help people in your community. Hold on to that spark; it will keep you motivated as you go through the difficult but gratifying years of medical school.

A World of Information Waits for You

Medical school opens up a world of complicated biological processes, interesting physical structures, and the complicated ways that health and illness affect each other. Learn about physiology (how the body works on the inside), pharmacology (drugs and how they work), and pathology (the changes that happen on a tiny and macro level when someone is sick). You will have a full understanding of the human body in both healthy and sick states as each new idea builds on the one before it.

Beyond Memorization: How to Develop Critical Thinking

Knowing a lot of facts is important, but learning how to be a good doctor takes more than that. Medical school teaches you how to think critically, which means you learn how to look at complicated situations, tell the difference between diagnoses, and make good clinical choices. Learn to look at each case like a mystery and use the patient's background, the results of the physical exam, and diagnostic tests to piece together clues that will help you make a correct diagnosis and a good treatment plan.

Learning How to Talk to People and Earn Their Trust

Not only does clinical understanding play a big role in providing excellent medical care, but so does clear communication. You'll learn how to clearly and briefly explain complicated medical ideas to your patients, which will help you build trust and a relationship with them. Active listening skills are just as important because they help you understand their worries, concerns, and healthcare goals. A good medical practice is built on strong relationships with its patients.

Accept Lifelong Learning: A Doctor's Promise

Medicine is a field that is always changing. Research, diagnostic tools, and healing methods are making huge steps forward at a rate that has never been seen before. A dedication to learning throughout life is an important part of this job. Learn to be curious in order to keep up with new developments, keep learning more, and change your practice to reflect the newest evidence-based medicine.

The Road Ahead: Difficulties and Progress

Going to medical school is a tough process. There will be times when you feel frustrated, nights when you stay up late studying, and the stress of important tests. There will be hard times, but there will also be amazing victories: the thrill of understanding a complicated idea, the satisfaction of making a patient feel better, and the friendships you make with other students who share your love for healing.

Do Not Forget Why You Began

When the path ahead seems too hard, remember what made you want to become a doctor in the first place. Think about how your work will affect the lives of your patients, how you'll help those in need, and how you'll make the world a better place. Use your desire to guide you and push you forward as you go through the exciting and life-changing years of medical school.

This chapter has given you a taste of the world that's to come. The chapters that follow will go into more detail about certain parts of your medical education. These will give you the information and tools you need to do well in this challenging but rewarding academic setting. Put your seat belt on, future doctor, and get ready for a great trip!

CHAPTER 2

HOW TO DEVELOP A GROWTH MINDSET

Love Challenges

Things that need to be done in order to become medical marvels are hard. From learning hard medical ideas to passing tough tests, the journey will definitely push you to your limits. Don't worry, brave student! The growth attitude is a powerful tool that you will learn about in this chapter.

Fixed vs. Growth: How to Understand the Way People Think

Imagine that two kids have to take a hard test. A person with a fixed mindset thinks that their intelligence is fixed and that failures show them what they can't do. The other person has a growth mindset, which means they see problems as chances to learn and improve. They think that if they work hard and don't give up, they can get smarter.

The Trap of the Fixed Mindset: A fixed mindset can really get in the way of your progress. It can make people give up when things get hard, not want to leave their safety zone, and afraid of failing.

Getting on board with the growth mindset: The good news? It is possible to develop a growth mindset! This chapter will talk about ways to:

Challenges as Stepping Stones: Instead of seeing problems as problems to be solved, learn to see them as chances to improve your skills and knowledge.

Celebrate Effort over Outcome: Value the journey as much as the goal and focus on how hard you work at learning.

Accept Feedback as Fuel: see helpful advice as a way to get better, not as a way to judge your worth.

How to Develop a Growth Mindset Strength:

This chapter isn't just about ideas; it's also about doing things! We'll give you tasks you can do right away to improve your growth mindset:

Put yourself to the test: Try something new and hard to get out of your comfort zone.

Re-frame your self-talk: fight negative beliefs about yourself with positive statements that stress your ability to grow.

Learn from Mistakes: Look at your mistakes and find ways to get better. Turn your mistakes into steps that will help you reach your goals.

Find inspiration by reading about great people who overcame problems by working hard and having a growth mindset.

Learning new things all the time is the only way to become a medical marvel. Once you have a growth attitude, problems will no longer seem like obstacles but rather chances to get better. Do not forget that the smartest people are not born that way; they are those who learn to love it and welcome the difficulties that help them grow. Having a growth attitude and being completely committed to your goals will help you get to where you want to be in medicine.

CHAPTER 3

UNLEASHING YOUR DRIVE

How to Learn for the Rest of Your Life

School for medicine is a journey, not a sprint. Due to the large amount of information you'll be exposed to, you'll need to be very motivated to get through difficult coursework, tough tests, and the lifelong learning that is expected of medical professionals. This chapter talks about the power of intrinsic drive, which can spark your desire to learn and give you the strength to keep going on your medical journey.

Beyond Grades: The Power of Self-Motivation

Some things, like grades and awards, can motivate you, but the real key to success in medical school is innate motivation, which is the desire to learn and grow because it makes you happy. Intrinsic motivation means that you want to learn for its own sake. This feeds your curiosity and pushes you to learn more about the interesting complexities of the human body and disease.

Keeping your fire burning: intrinsic drivers in medicine

There are a number of internal drivers that can spark your desire to keep learning in medicine:

The Search for Knowledge: A real interest in the human body and how it works can be a strong motivator. Enjoy the wonder of how organs work together, how diseases can mess up these systems, and how medical treatments can make people healthy again. Ask questions, learn more about things that interest you, and enjoy the thrill of finding. Think about how amazed you were when you first learned about how the immune system fights off germs or how the respiratory and circulatory systems work together.

The Will to Help Others: The main goal of medicine is to ease people's pain and make their lives better. Think about how you'll affect the lives of your future patients: how you'll comfort them during a tough diagnosis, how you'll give them hope as you guide them through treatment, and how your presence will improve their health. If you want to become a doctor, this should push you to learn all the information and skills you need to give great care. Just think about how good you'll feel when your knowledge and skills directly lead to better results for patients.

The Challenge of the Unknown: The human body is like a complicated puzzle, and medicine is full of secrets that have yet to be solved. Take pleasure in the task of dealing with complicated medical cases, the thrill of making different diagnoses, and the satisfaction of finding the right answer.

Every new task should be seen as a chance to learn more and get better at clinical reasoning. Think about how satisfying it is to figure out a very tough diagnosis by putting together clues from a patient's background, symptoms, and test results.

Learning for Life as a Journey, Not a Goal: Medical information is always changing. A lot of new findings, technological advances, and treatment breakthroughs happen all the time. Accept that learning throughout your life is a process, not a goal. Keep up with the latest research by being curious, and develop a love of learning that will help you in your medical job. Imagine that you are at the cutting edge of medical knowledge and know how to use the newest study to make care for patients better.

Tips for Getting Your Own Motivation to Grow

Here are some useful things you can do to keep your internal drive high:

Find Your Niche: Medicine is a very broad field, and there are many specialties and areas of interest. Try volunteering in a variety of clinical settings and different areas to find what you're truly passionate about. Focusing on a certain area of interest can make learning more interesting and important. You might be interested in the workings of the nervous system or the difficulties of emergency care.

Set Learning Goals: Don't just study for tests; make learning goals for yourself. Aim to get good at a certain skill, learn more about an interesting subject, or take on a tough case study. Having personal goals that go beyond marks or what other people expect of you makes you feel like you own your learning journey and have accomplished things. Make it your goal to learn more about a new medical technology being used in your area of interest, or push yourself to get a better grasp on a complicated bodily process.

Connect the Dots: Sometimes it can feel like there is too much medical information. Look for ways that different topics are related. What effect does physiology have on pathology? How do the rules of pharmacology affect choices about treatment? Knowing how medical information is linked together makes it more useful and unified. Make a mind map or other graphic aid to show how different areas of anatomy, biochemistry, and pharmacology are related.

Find a Mentor: Ask inspiring doctors or teachers who live by the idea of lifelong learning for advice. Their passion and commitment can inspire you, and having them as a mentor can help you learn a lot and feel supported as you go through your medical journey. Look for someone who is not only knowledgeable about the subject but also really loves it and loves sharing that love with people.

Celebrate Your Successes: No matter how small or big your growth is, you should be proud of it. Mastering a difficult idea, doing well on a tough test, or finishing a clinical rotation are all big accomplishments that should be celebrated. It's good to remember your successes because they make you want to keep doing great things. Take a moment to think about how far you've come, how much you've learned, and how hard you've worked on your trip.

In conclusion

In medicine, success depends on people being motivated for their own reasons. Using your natural curiosity, desire to help others, and love of learning to your advantage will make medical school a rewarding and enriching experience. Take on the challenges, be proud of your accomplishments, and start this lifelong path of learning with a desire to find out more and make the world a better place. The next part goes into detail about time management, which is an important skill for medical school students who have a lot of work to do.

Part 2

How to Get Good at Medical Knowledge

CHAPTER 4
MASTERING TIME MANAGEMENT
Taking on the Coursework

There is a huge amount of work to do in medical school, and it seems like there is always new information to learn. Don't worry, though! Learning how to handle your time well will help you get through this difficult academic journey quickly and easily. This chapter gives you strong tools to master the course material, get the most done, and find time for a balanced life outside of school.

Understanding the Problem of Time Management

It's hard to keep track of time when you're in medical school. It can be hard to balance classes, labs, study groups, extracurricular activities, and your personal life. Here are some problems that medical students often have with managing their time:

Information Overload: There is so much information about medicine that it can be overwhelming. There are a lot of complicated details in textbooks and teachers teach complicated ideas every day. It can be very hard to remember everything.

Competing Priorities: It can be hard to find a balance between schoolwork, personal health, social life, and sleep. It's easy for the stresses of medical school to spill over into weekends and nights, leaving little time for fun, hobbies, or spending time with family and friends.

Delaying: It can be very tempting to wait until the last minute to do something, especially if you have a lot of work to do. This often causes students to cram, miss deadlines, and feel stressed out for no reason, which hurts their grades.

Distractions: We are constantly being bombarded with distractions in this digital age, which makes it hard to concentrate on tough study sessions. Notifications from social media, emails, and the constant desire to check our phones can make it hard to focus and get things done.

Getting better at managing your time

Before you start using specific strategies, you should have a growth attitude about managing your time. How to change your point of view:

Time management is a skill that can be polished and improved over time. It's not something that you're naturally good at. It takes experience, dedication, and a willingness to try out different methods to find the ones that work best for you, just like any other skill.

Take advantage of structure and planning: Don't be afraid to make plans and routines. Structure is what makes success possible. Even if something unexpected happens, having a plan lets you change your direction without getting too stressed out.

Keep your eye on progress instead of perfection. You will have failures and days when your best efforts don't quite cut it. For example, you might not give yourself enough time to study, or you might get lost on social media. The important thing is to learn from these mistakes, change how you do things as needed, and keep your eye on steady progress instead of setting impossible daily goals.

Celebrate Your Success: No matter how big or small your success is, you should be proud of it. It's a victory when you finish a particularly hard chapter, do well on a difficult test, or even just stick to your study plan for a week. Seeing how far you've come reinforces good behavior and inspires you to keep working toward your school goals.

Tips for Medical Students on How to Manage Their Time

Create Your Own Schedule: Make a weekly or monthly plan that sets aside specific times for classes, tests, study sessions, meals, sleep, and fun activities. Be realistic and plan for extra time in case something unexpected comes up or you need to catch up on work you missed. Use planners, scheduling apps, or bullet journals to stay organized and keep track of your responsibilities visually.

Set priorities without mercy: not all jobs are equal. Figure out which jobs are the most important for each day and put them in order of importance. Techniques like the Eisenhower Matrix can help you sort jobs into groups based on how important and how quickly they need to be done. This will help you focus on what's most important. Important and urgent jobs, like studying for an upcoming test, should come before checking social media or going to a club meeting that isn't necessary.

Set aside time to study: Don't depend on random cramming sessions the night before a test. Set aside time each week for focused study sessions where you will go over class notes, practice answering problem-solving questions, and make sure you fully understand what you are learning. Active learning methods, like making flashcards, spaced repetition, and summarizing important ideas in your own words, are much better for long-term memory retention than idly reading textbooks again and again.

Active learning methods should be used instead of rote memory. In some areas of medicine, you need to be able to remember facts, but this doesn't always lead to a deep understanding of complicated ideas. Use active learning techniques like spaced repetition, writing your own summaries of key ideas, and making flashcards to help you remember and understand what you're learning. In a study group, teaching someone else about an idea can help you understand it better yourself.

Reduce Distractions: Turn off messages on your phone, find a quiet place to study, and think about using website blockers to cut down on distractions while you're concentrating. Tell your family and friends when you need to study so that they don't bother you. If background noise is really getting in the way of your work, you should get noise-canceling headphones.

Get together with other people to study. Working together is a great way to learn. You might want to form a study group with friends who want to learn as much as you do and are dedicated to working hard. Talk about hard topics, test each other on important ideas, and explain ideas to each other. Teaching someone else about a concept helps you understand it better and gives you access to new ideas and ways of learning. But make sure that your study group stays on task and gets things done. Do not let social events take over your study time and distract you.

Use the tools your school provides. For example, many medical schools offer tutoring centers, workshops on how to manage your time and study, and access to online learning materials. You should not be afraid to use these tools to help you learn more and solve any problems you may be having.

Plan breaks and make sleep a priority. Staying up all night to study may seem like a good idea at first, but it will hurt you in the long run. Sleep is very important for your brain's ability to think clearly and remember things. Aim to get at least 7-8 hours of good sleep every night. Take breaks during the day to keep your mind fresh and avoid getting burned out. Do something relaxing, like deep breathing or meditation, or do a short burst of physical activity to calm down and get ready for the next day.

Don't be afraid to say "no." Medical school is hard, but you don't have to do everything by yourself. Learn how to politely say no to requests that would make your life harder or put your health at risk. Put your health and academic obligations first, and don't be afraid to delegate chores or reschedule social events when you need to.

Keeping your life in balance is important. School is important, but ignoring your physical and mental health can hurt you. Set aside time to do the things you enjoy, like relaxing, exercising, spending time with family and friends, or exploring hobbies. Having a balanced life lowers stress, sharpens your focus, and promotes your general health, all of which will help you do better in school.

In conclusion

Time management is one of the most important skills you need to do well in medical school. By having a growth mindset, using these strategies, and putting your health first, you'll be able to master the course material, handle the heavy workload, and feel ready for the exciting journey ahead when you finish. Don't forget that managing your time is an ongoing process. As you find the best strategies for you, try new things, make changes to your approach as needed, and enjoy your growth. Your commitment to hard work and learning new things all the time will help you get through medical school and start a rewarding job in medicine.

CHAPTER 5
STRATEGIES FOR ACTIVE LEARNING
Getting Involved with the Material

There is so much information about medicine that it can be confusing at times. Passive learning, like rereading textbooks or idly underlining notes, can make you feel safe, but the only way to really understand and remember something is to actively work with it. This chapter goes over a bunch of useful active learning methods that will help you go from being a passive information consumer to a medical knowledge master.

Why it's Important to Learn Actively

Passive learning can make you feel good about what you've learned, but it usually leads to a shallow knowledge and a short-lived memory. Here are some ways that active learning can make your time in medical school better:

Better understanding: interacting with the information in a way that goes beyond memorization leads to a deeper understanding. Think about the difference between reading about the heart's structure and building a 3D model of it with clay or modeling tools. Making something causes you to see how things fit together in space, find important structures, and solidify your understanding in a way that reading something can't.

Better Memory Retention: Active learning methods are very good at fighting the "forgetting curve," which is the natural tendency to forget things over time. Think about what the difference is between actively testing yourself with flashcards or practice questions and passively going over a chapter on pharmacology again. Active recall makes the neural connections that hold knowledge stronger, which makes it easier to find when you need it. During a clinical shift, you might need to remember a certain drug interaction. If you've practiced finding that information with flashcards, it will be much easier to find than if you just read the chapter again a few times.

Getting Better at Critical Thinking: Active learning does more than just help you remember facts; it also gives you the critical thinking skills you need to diagnose and treat people. Think about what it would be like to actively analyze a case study to choose between possible diagnoses based on the information given versus passively remembering a list of symptoms for a certain disease. Active learning helps you learn how to think critically, compare information from different sources, and use what you've learned in real life.

This is exactly what you'll need to do when you're a doctor and you have to deal with complicated cases.

Building Confidence and Motivation: Working hard on the subject and understanding difficult ideas is a satisfying process that makes you feel better about your own abilities. Solving a hard practice problem or explaining a medical idea to a peer in a way that helps them understand is a powerful motivator that feeds your natural desire to keep learning.

Techniques for Active Learning for Medical Marvels

If you want to learn more about how to use active learning to your advantage, here are some studies tips:

Self-Tests and Practice Questions: Use notes, practice problems from textbooks and online sources, or old test questions to test yourself on a regular basis. Do not simply accept the answer; instead, take the time to explain your thought process in your own words. This process of active remembering improves memory and shows you what you need to learn more about.

Concept Mapping and Mind Maps: Don't get stuck in taking notes in a straight line. Instead, use concept maps or mind maps to organize knowledge visually. These tools help you see how different ideas are related, which helps you understand and remember things better. As you make these maps, you might want to use different colors for different topics or pictures to help you remember what you saw.

Explanation and Teaching: One of the best ways to make sure you understand something is to explain it to a friend or imagine yourself teaching it to a patient in a way that they can easily understand. Writing down information in your own words pushes you to figure out where you might not know as much and improve your explanations to make them clear. This is a powerful way to not only improve your own learning but also improve your communication skills, which are necessary for getting along with patients.

Case Studies and Clinical Applications: By breaking down case studies, you can put yourself in real-life situations. Look at the symptoms, diagnostic tests, treatment methods, and possible results. This fills in the gaps between what we know in theory and how we use it in patient care. Look for case studies that cover a variety of medical situations. This will help you get a full picture of how medical knowledge is used to make clinical decisions.

Collaborative learning and group discussions: Get together with people who share your interests to study and talk about tough topics, test each other, and argue about different points of view. When you explain ideas to others, listen to different points of view, and work through problems with others, you gain a deeper knowledge and experience different ways of learning.

The Feynman Technique: Imagine teaching a medical idea to someone who doesn't know much about it, like a child. Making yourself break down information into clear, easy terms helps you understand it better and shows you where you might not know enough. The Feynman Technique is a great way to find out what you don't know and make sure you can explain even the most complicated medical ideas in a way that other people can understand.

Making The Most of Your Active Learning

It's not enough to just throw techniques at the wall and hope something sticks when you're active learning. To get the most out of your active learning, here are some tips:

Match the Method to the Content: There are various ways to learn that work better with various kinds of knowledge. You can use flashcards to remember the names of drugs or the structures of the body, but idea maps might help you understand how complex physiological processes work.

Do not do all of your active learning tasks in one long session. Instead, spread them out over time. To improve long-term memory, use spaced repetition, which means going over knowledge more and more far apart.

Think About What You've Learned: After using an active learning approach, think about how well it worked for you. Did it help you understand better? Did it show any gaps in your knowledge? Always think about how you're learning and change your methods to get the best results.

Take on the Challenge: Active learning may require more work than inactive studying, but the benefits are great. Take on the task and see it as a chance to learn more and boost your intelligence.

In conclusion

You'll go from being a passive consumer of information to a master of medical knowledge if you use active learning techniques in medical school. You'll not only do well on your tests, but you'll also learn how to think critically and solve problems, which will make you a great doctor. Don't forget that active learning is a process, not a goal. Try out different methods until you find the one that works best for you, and enjoy the journey of learning that lies ahead.

CHAPTER 6
GETTING MORE KNOWLEDGE
Textbooks, Lectures, and More

The medical school program calls for a wide range of learning tools. To help you learn and remember more, this chapter gives you a complete set of tools and tells you how to use textbooks, classes, and many other sources in the best way possible.

The Textbook: The Basis of Medical Understanding

Textbooks are the most important thing you can use to learn about medicine. To get the most out of them, do the following:

Choosing the Right Textbooks: Buy high-quality, well-known textbooks that professors or upperclassmen suggest. Think about things like how well the writing is organized and whether there are any helpful pictures or tables. Don't be afraid to look at more than one guide on the same subject to get a complete picture. Look for suggestions from teachers who are known for being experts in certain subjects, and use what they say to choose relevant extra readings.

Active Reading Strategies: Don't just read it again! Active reading methods include underlining important ideas, writing your own summaries of what you've read, and making notes in the margins that make you think of questions or make connections to other ideas. By making notes in your textbooks, you can make a unique study guide that fits the way you learn and shows you what you need to learn more about.

Connect Textbooks and Lectures: Don't think of lectures and textbooks as two different things. You can use your material to learn more about ideas you've heard in class, and the other way around. Look for information that goes along with what you already know and examples that help you understand better. Textbooks can give you a broad overview of a subject, but lectures can give you teachers' unique points of view, clinical anecdotes, and insights that show you how medical knowledge can be used in real life.

Lectures: The Keys to Gaining Deeper Understanding

Professors can go into more detail about difficult topics, talk about their professional experience, and answer your questions during lectures. Here are some tips to get the most out of your lecture:

Get Ready: Read the appropriate chapter of your textbook ahead of time to get a feel for the main ideas. This will help you follow the lesson better and figure out what parts need more explanation. If you're ready for class, you'll be able to ask more targeted questions that will help you understand the subject better during the lecture.

Active listening means you don't just take notes. Engage with what you're hearing and write down not only facts but also ideas, questions that make you think, and links to what you've already read in your literature. Look for ways to relate what the teacher is talking about to what you already know and have experienced. This will not only help you understand better, but it will also make learning more fun.

Besides taking notes, recording classes (as long as you get permission first) can be helpful. Don't count on recordings alone, though. Actively take notes during the lesson, and then listen to the recording again to fill in any blanks and make sure you understand. Pay close attention to how the professor stresses certain ideas; this can help you figure out how important they are for tests or future clinical practice.

Getting outside of textbooks and lectures to broaden your horizons

There is a lot more to learn about medicine than what you can find in textbooks and classes. Here is a great trove of extra materials that will help you learn more:

Online Resources: Look into good online resources like educational websites for doctors, online libraries, and educational apps. To help people understand better, these sites often have animations, self-testing tools, and interactive parts. Find online tools that go along with your textbooks and class notes. But make sure you check the source's reliability before adding the information to your knowledge base.

Medical Journals: Read reputable medical journals to learn about the newest medical study. Start with articles about things you've learned in class and work your way up to themes that interest you more. Some medical journals require paid subscriptions, but many schools give their students access to large online databases of medical journals. At first, it might be hard to read research papers, but with practice, you'll learn how to think critically about the research methods and combine the results to better understand complicated medical topics.

Clinical Correlation Resources: Use resources that show how medical knowledge can be used in the real world to bridge the gap between theory and practice. Look for collections of case studies, websites that show real-life patient situations, or textbooks that are designed to help you make clinical connections. When you use clinical correlation resources, you can see how the things you're learning in school can be used to diagnose and treat patients. This makes learning more meaningful and helps you understand how medical science is used in real life.

Cadaver labs and anatomy models: learning by doing is very important in medical school. By letting you see anatomical structures in three dimensions, cadaver labs give you a unique chance to learn more about the human body. You can also use anatomy models to help you learn more outside of textbooks and improve your sense of space. Working with cadavers or anatomical models is a hands-on way to learn about body structures that can be much more useful than just memorizing pictures from a book.

Working together to learn is a great way to get things done. Get together with people who share your interests to study and talk about hard topics, test each other, and help each other understand what they're reading. Teaching others about an idea not only helps you understand it better yourself, but it also lets you see things from other people's points of view and learning styles. Find study partners whose skills and weaknesses are similar to yours. This will make the classroom more interesting.

Opportunities for mentoring and shadowing: Ask experienced medical workers for help. Follow doctors around as they do their rounds, watch how they talk to patients, and ask smart questions. As a mentor, someone who is passionate about medicine can give you advice on your job and give you valuable insights into how the medical field really works. Some jobs let you "shadow" a doctor so you can see how their medical knowledge is used in real life. This gives you a look into their daily life.

Mnemonic Devices and Flashcards: Utilize mnemonic devices and flashcards to remember challenging terms, drug names, or anatomical structures. Create your own mnemonics that are personally important and engaging, or utilize pre-made flashcards from reputable sources. Mnemonics and flashcards can be helpful for rote memorization, but ensure you don't depend solely on them for deeper understanding.

Practice Makes Perfect: Solidify your learning by applying your knowledge to practice tasks. Look for practice questions at the end of textbook chapters, utilize online question banks, or participate in mock exams offered by student groups. Regularly testing your knowledge identifies areas needing improvement, reinforces key concepts, and prepares you for the types of questions you might face on exams.

In conclusion

Building your knowledge arsenal goes beyond simply collecting information. It's about creating a diverse learning ecosystem that caters to your unique learning style and optimizes information retention. By using textbooks, lectures, and many other tools well, you'll go from being a new medical student to a well-equipped learner who is ready to start a lifelong journey of discovery in the fascinating field of medicine. Remember that the key to success is not just learning things, but also having the drive, interest, and passion to keep learning and growing throughout your medical job.

Part 3

Improving What You Remember and Can Remember

CHAPTER 7
THE POWER OF PRACTICE
More Than Just Reading

When you go to medical school, you learn a lot about the theory behind medicine. Deep dive into complicated biological processes, master the complexity of the human body, and learn everything you need to know about different diseases. But real success comes from using what you've learned in real life. This chapter talks about the different kinds of practice and how important they are. It gives you the tools to turn your academic knowledge into useful skills that will help you become a well-rounded doctor.

Why practice is important in medicine

Textbooks and lectures are great ways to learn, but medicine is a very hands-on job. **Here are some reasons why it's important to actively practice what you know**:

How to Close the Gap Between Knowledge and Skill: Knowing the theory is only the beginning. By using what you've learned, you can improve important clinical skills like doing a physical check, figuring out what diagnostic tests mean, and talking to patients in a clear way. For example, reading about the different heart sounds in a guidebook is more useful when you use a stethoscope to listen to a patient's heart and learn to tell the difference between normal and abnormal sounds.

Increasing Your Confidence and Skill: Your confidence and skill will grow as you use what you've learned in real life situations. Seeing how your actions affect patient care makes you feel good about what you've done and encourages you to keep learning and improving as a future doctor. You'll feel more at ease and skilled in a variety of clinical situations the more you practice basic skills.

Improving your ability to think critically and solve problems: In real life, medical cases are rarely like those in textbooks. You'll learn how to look at complicated situations, gather relevant data, come up with different diagnoses, and make choices about patient care that are based on good information. Using what you've learned to solve real-life medical problems improves your ability to think critically and solve problems. This prepares you for the unknowns that come with clinical work.

Improving Communication and Social Skills: In medicine, it's very important to be able to communicate clearly. You can get better at getting along with patients, listening to their worries, and explaining complicated medical ideas in a way that they can understand by practicing. Role-playing games with peers or "standardized patients" can help you get better at interacting with people in real life. They can also help you improve your communication skills and get better at telling people bad news or complicated diagnoses with compassion and empathy.

Different Ways to Practice

Medicine is practiced in places other than hospitals and clinics. There are a number of ways to improve your skills and get from theory to practice:

Sessions in the lab: Sessions in the lab give you a safe and controlled place to practice important technical skills like drawing blood, stitching, and running medical tests. During these classes, you can get better at dexterity, hand-eye coordination, and using different kinds of medical equipment while being supervised by trained professionals.

Exercise Labs: These days, medical schools often have high-tech exercise labs with mannequins that act and react like real people. You can practice medical procedures, handle emergencies, and handle difficult clinical situations in these rooms, which are safe and well-controlled. Before working with real patients, simulation labs are a great way to get practice and improve your skills.

Encounters with Standardized Patients: Standardized patients are actors who have been taught to show certain medical conditions and symptoms. This gives you a chance to practice taking histories, doing physical exams, and talking to people in a real-life setting. Getting feedback on your communication, bedside manner, and clinical reasoning from trained facilitators can help you figure out what you need to work on and boost your confidence for when you deal with patients in the real world.

Clinical training: The best way to learn by doing in medical school is through clinical training. These rotations put you in real-life healthcare settings where you can use what you've learned to care for patients while being supervised by more experienced doctors. During each rotation, you will have the chance to see how patients connect with each other, take part in physical exams, and help make treatment plans. Clinical rotations are a great way to improve your clinical skills, build your professional personality, and find out what area of medicine interests you the most.

Case studies and problem-solving activities: Looking at real or made-up medical cases helps you use what you've learned in the classroom to solve tough clinical issues. Talking about these cases with classmates or teachers helps with critical thinking, developing the ability to tell the difference between diagnoses, and coming up with treatment plans that are based on evidence. You will be able to handle real-life clinical situations with more confidence after doing these tasks.

In conclusion

Practice is the most important part of turning medical information into useful skills. You'll bridge the gap between theory and practice, gain confidence and competence, and develop the critical thinking and speaking skills you need to do well as a doctor if you actively participate in different types of practice. Take advantage of every chance to use your skills, learn from your mistakes, and keep trying to get better. Remember that you will always be learning in medicine. You are changing from a medical student to a well-rounded, caring, and skilled doctor. Enjoy the challenges, enjoy your progress, and delight in the process.

CHAPTER 8

MEMORY MAGIC

How to Remember Things for a Long Time

You are constantly being flooded with information in medical school. It goes on: anatomy, physiology, medicine, biochemistry, and so on. It is very important to remember this huge amount of information so that you can do well on your tests and, more importantly, so that you can confidently use it in clinical situations in the real world. This chapter talks about strong memory techniques that can help you store information in your long-term memory. This will help you do well in school and learn what you need to know to become a good doctor.

The Study of How We Remember and Keep Things

Knowing how memory works is the first step in using successful techniques for remembering things. In simpler terms, here's what it means:

Short-term memory is the short-term storage space in your brain that holds a small amount of knowledge for a short time. It's like a notepad in your head. If you don't constantly practice or consolidate what you remember in short-term memory, it fades quickly.

Long-Term Memory: This is where details are saved for a long time. The goal of good learning techniques is to move information from your short-term memory to your long-term memory so that you can remember it for a long time.

Encoding: is the process of putting data into a form that your brain can fully understand and remember. The memory trace is stronger when encoding techniques work well, which increases the chances that the knowledge will be stored in long-term memory.

Retrieval: means being able to get to and remember information that has been saved when you need it. Active learning and spaced repetition help with retrieval by making the memory pathways that link to the knowledge stronger.

Moving from learning passively to learning actively

In medicine, rote learning, or just cramming facts into your short-term memory, doesn't help you remember them for long periods of time. This approach might help you pass a test, but it won't give you the deep understanding you need to work as a doctor. Here are some ways to help you remember things better and store them more deeply, turning you from a passive information user into an active learner:

Learning by doing: Don't just read your studies over and over again. Use active learning methods to get involved with the subject. Write down the main ideas in your own words, as if you were describing them to a patient or a classmate who is having trouble with the subject. This causes you to explain things clearly, which helps you understand them better and strengthens the memory trace.

Spaced repetition is a way to remember things for a long time. Going over the same information more and more far apart makes it easier to find later. In this case, flashcards that use timed repetition can be very helpful. Start by going over new knowledge often. As your memory gets better, slowly increase the time between reviews. This method works like the natural forgetfulness curve and makes sure you go over important ideas again before you forget them completely.

Elaborative Encoding: Make Connections: Link new information to what you already know. Think about how this new idea is related to diseases you already know about, bodily functions you understand, or medicines that work in similar ways. Making mental connections, similarities, or stories between new information and things you already know helps you understand it better and remember it. For example, instead of remembering a long list of foot bones, picture how they are put together and how they work as a weight-bearing arch. This will help you understand biomechanics better.

Create Shortcuts: Mnemonics are memory tools that help you store and retrieve information. They come in the form of acronyms, rhymes, or songs. Like, "PEMDAS" is a phrase that helps people remember the order of math operations: parentheses, exponents, multiplication and division from left to right, and addition and subtraction from left to right. You can make your own mnemonics or use ones that are already made for medical terms to help you remember things like drug names, side effects, or diagnostic criteria.

Use Diagrams and Charts for Visual Learning: Diagrams, charts, and flowcharts can help people who learn best by seeing things. Drawing pictures of body parts, making flowcharts to show how the body works, or using mind maps to clearly organize complicated ideas can help you remember and find information. The way your brain processes and stores knowledge is different when you look at these pictures.

Making the most of your learning space to help you remember

Your mental and physical health have a big effect on how well you can learn and remember things. Here are some ideas for making the best learning space that helps you remember things:

Cut down on distractions: Find a place to study that is quiet and doesn't have any noise, trash, or social media alerts. Turn off your phone, let your family or roommates know that you need to study alone, and use website blockers to avoid the temptations of surfing the web. Distractions split up your focus, making it hard to process information correctly.

Prioritize Sleep to Strengthen Your Memories: Your brain works best when you're well-rested. Aim to get at least 7-8 hours of good sleep every night. Not getting enough sleep makes it harder to concentrate, store knowledge, and link memories together for long-term use. Your brain works on and improves the memories it made while you were awake while you sleep.

Maintain a Healthy Lifestyle for Best Brain Function: Living a healthy life gives your brain power and helps you remember things. Make sure you get enough fruits, veggies, whole grains, and lean protein in your diet. Regular exercise increases blood flow to the brain, which helps it work better. Deal with your stress by relaxing with deep breathing or meditation. Stress can make it harder to make and remember memories. Being mindful of your physical and mental health is important for learning and remembering things.

Regularly Test Yourself: Don't wait until the night before an exam to see how well you remember things. Set up self-tests with practice questions, flashcards, or old test papers to use throughout the term. Actively getting information from your memory makes the memory trace stronger and shows you what you need to go over again. You might want to get together with some friends to study and quiz each other on important ideas. Teaching someone else about an idea helps you remember it and makes your own learning stronger.

In conclusion

Memory methods that work are not magic tricks; they are powerful tools that can help you learn more in medical school. You can go from being a passive consumer of information to an active learner who can store information for long-term retention if you understand the science behind memory, use active learning methods, and make the most of your study space. Remember that a good memory is essential for success in medicine. It will help you do well in school and give great care to your patients in the future. Take these tips, try them out, and see which ones work best for you. As a doctor, you will always be learning new things. In the next chapter, we'll talk about critical thinking, which is an important skill for making clinical decisions and reasoning in medicine.

CHAPTER 9
WORKING TOGETHER TO LEARN
Teaching and Learning With Other People

It's hard to get through medical school, but you don't have to do it by yourself. Studying and learning with other people, also known as collaborative learning, has many benefits. It can improve your classroom experience, help you understand difficult medical ideas better, and get you ready for the collaborative nature of clinical practice. This part talks about the benefits of working with others to learn and gives you tips on how to make good study groups, use online resources, and get the most out of your interactions with classmates to learn.

The Good Things About Learning Together

Working together to learn is more than just studying in the same room. It's about working together with your classmates to build information and get a better grasp of the subject.

This is how group learning can help you:

Better Memory: When you explain an idea to a classmate, you have to do more than just memorize it; you have to be able to articulate it properly. This process helps you understand better by making you break down difficult topics into easier terms. Talking about these issues with friends who come from different backgrounds helps you see things from different points of view and improves your understanding of the material from different sides. Imagine trying to explain the Krebs cycle to a friend who has a hard time with it. By training them, you have to figure out the most important steps, explain how they fit together, and clear up any underlying confusions. All of these things help you understand things better.

Better Problem-Solving Skills: Working on tough problems with other people in a study group setting helps people think critically, come up with ideas, and come up with creative solutions. Group talks help people see things from different points of view, spot possible biases, and think of other possible explanations. This ability to work together to solve problems will directly apply to the clinical setting, where you'll be expected to diagnose and create treatment plans for patients with complicated medical conditions with the help of nurses, specialists, and other medical workers.

Getting better at talking to people and getting along with them: In medicine, good conversation is very important. Collaborative learning gives you a chance to improve your ability to communicate clearly, listen carefully, and respectfully present and support your ideas. You will learn how to explain difficult medical ideas in a way that your friends and future patients can understand. You can also improve your active listening skills in group discussions by paying full attention to your peers and recognizing what they have to say. As you deal with differences or different points of view in your study group, you'll learn how to respectfully defend your ideas while also considering other points of view. This is a very important skill for working with others and getting along with patients.

Encouragement and Help: Studying with other people can really help you stay motivated, especially since medical school is very hard. Sharing the ups and downs of medical school with people who are going through the same things can help build community and make the journey seem less scary. You can get through hard times and enjoy your successes more easily if you know you're not alone in your struggles and have people you can lean on.

Being exposed to different ways of learning: Everyone has their own way of learning. One big benefit of collaborative learning is that you get to know peers who are good and bad at different things. A friend who is great at making diagrams or flowcharts to show how physiological processes work could help someone who learns best by seeing. Auditory learners might learn a lot from talking with friends who can clearly explain ideas. People who learn best through movement might enjoy group events where they act out case studies or physically show how body parts work. Working with a broad group will expose you to different ways of learning and help you find new ways to understand difficult medical ideas.

How to Make Study Groups Work and More

Here are some useful tips to get the most out of your relationships with peers now that you know why collaborative learning is good:

Find Peers Who Are Like You: Look for peers who share your learning goals, work ethic, and desire to learn together. A group of people from different backgrounds, each with their own skills and weaknesses, can help create a well-rounded learning space. You might want to form a study group with two to four classmates who are mentally challenging you and with whom you feel comfortable.

Set Ground Rules and Plan Your Sessions: Talk about and agree on the ground rules for your study group meetings. This could mean making clear goals for each session (like going over a certain chapter again, practicing problem-solving questions, or studying for an upcoming test), listening to what everyone has to say, staying focused, and sticking to the time you agreed to. Active learning methods, such as case studies, practice questions, and group talks, will help you keep everyone interested and on track with your learning goal.

Use online collaboration tools. In this digital age, there are many online platforms that can help people learn together without having to be in the same room. You can share resources, ask peers questions, and have discussions without being online at the same time using discussion forums or online collaborative whiteboards. It can be very helpful to use online tools to organize your schedule, share notes or summaries, and stay in touch with peers between meetings.

In conclusion

Working with other people to learn is a useful method that can help you do well in medical school and become a well-rounded doctor. You'll not only better understand complicated medical information by interacting with your peers, explaining ideas, taking part in group talks, and using online tools, but you'll also improve your communication, interpersonal, and problem-solving skills. Remember that working together well is an important part of clinical practice. To provide the best care for patients, healthcare workers must be able to work well with others.

Collaborative learning helped you learn a lot and make friends in medical school. It will also help you when you start working with other people in clinical practice. Take advantage of the chance to learn from and help your classmates, and let's go on this path of personal and intellectual growth together.

Part 4

Habits for Well-Rounded Success Outside of School

CHAPTER 10

TAKING CARE OF YOURSELF

Keeping Your Mind and Body Healthy

It takes a long time to become a medical wonder. The hard work in class and the constant stress can hurt your mental and physical health. This chapter teaches you important ways to take care of yourself so that you can handle the tasks of medical school while putting your health and happiness first.

The Link Between Mind and Body in Medical School

If the cup is empty, you can't pour. Putting your physical and mental health first isn't a nice-to-have; it's a must for doing well in school and being successful in the long run. Here's how these two things are deeply connected:

Physical health affects mental health. For example, regular exercise, a healthy diet, and enough sleep are all important for staying focused, concentrating, and emotionally strong. It's harder to deal with stress, stay focused, and remember things when you're physically tired. Many research studies have clearly linked being active with better brain functions like memory, attention, and processing speed. In contrast, not getting enough sleep on a regular basis can make you anxious and depressed, which can make it harder to handle the responsibilities of medical school.

Mental health affects physical health. For example, long-term worry, anxiety, and not getting enough sleep can weaken your immune system, making you more likely to get sick. Hormones that cause stress, like cortisol, can damage your body and make you more likely to get long-term illnesses like diabetes and heart disease. Putting mental health practices like meditation and relaxation at the top of your list can make your physical health much better by lowering stress hormones and encouraging a healthy inflammatory reaction.

Putting together a base for physical health

Feed Your Body: A healthy meal full of fruits, vegetables, whole grains, and lean protein will fuel your brain and body. Stay away from processed foods, too much sugar, and bad fats that can make you tired and hurt your brain. If you plan your meals and snacks ahead of time, you can make healthy choices throughout the day and avoid reaching for unhealthy food at the vending machine when you have to study for a long time. Talk to a nutritionist about making a custom meal plan that will give you the most energy and help your brain work better.

Move Your Body: Doing regular exercise can help you deal with stress and improve your happiness. Aim to work out at a reasonable level for at least 30 minutes most days of the week. Whether it's going to the gym, dance class, or taking a fast walk outside, find things you love doing. Endorphins are natural mood boosters that fight worry and anxiety. Being active also improves the quality of your sleep, which is another important part of your physical and mental health. Moving around for short periods of time during the day can be helpful. Do jumping jacks during a study break, take the stairs instead of the elevator, or sign up for an online exercise class. All of these things will make you healthier and stronger.

Put sleep first. Aim for 7-8 hours of good sleep every night. Set a regular sleep time and make a relaxing routine for bedtime to get restful sleep that improves your health, focus, and memory. Set up a relaxing routine before bed that tells your body it's time to unwind. This could mean doing something like taking a warm bath, reading a book, or relaxing by doing things like deep breathing or meditation. Stay away from screens for at least an hour before bed, because the blue light they give off can mess up your sleep cycle.

Listen to Your Body: Learn to read your body's signs when it's hungry, tired, or stressed. Schedule time to relax and take breaks when you need to. Also, don't be afraid to ask for help or share work when it gets too much. Even though your body is a great machine, it has its boundaries. Trying to do too much will only make you tired and hurt your general performance. Watch out for warning signs like headaches, stomachaches, or trouble focusing. These things might be telling you that you need to take a break, recharge, and then go back to studying with more energy and focus.

Taking care of your mental health

Mindfulness and Meditation: Adding deep breathing techniques or meditation to your daily routine can help you become more mindful. These methods can help you deal with stress, concentrate better, and feel better emotionally. Training your attention to be in the present moment without judging it is what mindfulness meditation is all about. You can learn to calm down and quiet your mind in the middle of medical school by paying attention to your breath and how your body feels. Online and app guides for guided meditation are easy to find and can help you start this practice.

Positive Self-Talk: Fight your negative thoughts and learn to have a growth attitude. Instead of dwelling on setbacks, see them as chances to learn and enjoy your wins, no matter how small. The voice inside our heads can be very harsh, but it doesn't have to run our lives. Use positive affirmations to fight negative thoughts and to remember yourself of your strengths and what you've already done well. Think about yourself achieving and focus on the good things that are happening along the way. Saying nice things to yourself can really help your confidence, drive, and toughness.

Get help: Don't hold your feelings inside. Tell someone about your problems, like a therapist, family member, friend, or teacher. Having a strong network of support is important for dealing with stress and keeping your mental health in good shape. It can make a huge difference to know that people care about you and are willing to listen. You might want to join a support group for medical students. There, you can meet other students who understand the stresses and problems you're going through. Also, if you're having trouble with anxiety, sadness, or any other mental health issue, don't be afraid to get help from a therapist or counselor.

Maintain a Good Work-Life Balance: Plan time for fun things you like to do outside of school. Make time for things that make you happy and help you relax, like spending time with family and friends, doing hobbies, or just reading a good book. A good work-life mix is important to keep your motivation up while you are in medical school and avoid burnout. Just like your body needs rest and good food to work at its best, your mind does too. Plan time for fun things that will help you relax and recharge so that you can go back to studying feeling focused and refreshed.

Enjoy the Journey: Medical school is hard work that pays off in the end. There will be problems, setbacks, and times when you question your own abilities. But don't lose sight of the bigger picture: your love of medicine and the amazing job path that lies ahead. Enjoy the process of becoming a medical marvel, remember to celebrate your growth and learn from your mistakes.

In conclusion

It's not a sign of weakness to put your physical and mental health first; it's a sign of power. Developing healthy habits, getting help, and keeping a good work-life balance will give you the strength and health you need to do well in medical school and beyond. Remember that taking care of yourself is the best thing you can do for your future as a caring and successful healthcare worker.

CHAPTER 11
PUTTING TOGETHER STRONG SUPPORT SYSTEMS
Family, Friends, and Mentors

Medical school can be too much to handle with its tough classes, constant stress, and mental ups and downs. Dealing with these problems takes a strong support system, or a group of people who give you support, advice, and a sense of belonging as you go through medical school. This chapter talks about how having strong relationships with friends, family, and teachers can help your health and resilience.

How Important It Is to Have Plenty of Support

School for medicine is a journey, not a sprint. A strong support system is like a cheering section, a safety net, and a source of motivation during this difficult but gratifying process. **This is how having a helpful network helps you:**

Much less stress and anxiety: Knowing that people care about you and understand the stresses you're under can make you feel a lot better. Talking about your problems with someone you trust can help you deal with your feelings in a healthy way and see things from a different point of view. Keeping your feelings inside can make you tired and make it harder to handle the responsibilities of school. A supportive network gives you a safe place to let off steam, enjoy wins, and get support when things are tough.

Better motivation and focus: Having a support system can be like having your own personal cheerleader, encouraging you to keep going when things get tough and celebrating your successes. Having a group of people who believe in you can make all the difference when you're having a hard time with an idea or a test result that makes you feel down. As you work toward your goals, they can help you stay focused on the bigger picture—your love of medicine and the job you want to have in the future.

Better mental and physical health: Medical students often feel stressed out when they are alone or lonely, but having strong social ties can help. Research has shown that having friends and family around can lower blood pressure, boost the immune system, and even help people live longer. Being part of a supportive network makes you feel like you belong and improves your emotional health, both of which can have a good effect on your physical health and overall resilience. The other way around, long-term worry and loneliness can hurt your body and mind, making it even harder to handle the demands of medical school.

Help and Advice: Mentors with a lot of experience or upperclassmen can give you great advice on how to handle the academic and social life of medical school. They can talk about their experiences, such as the best ways to study and handle time, and give helpful tips on how to balance schoolwork with personal well-being. Mentors can also help you with your job by showing you different specialties and guiding you to find paths that match your interests and skills.

Putting together a support group

You don't have to limit your support system to just one type of person. Here's how to build good relationships with different people:

Friends and Classmates: Talk to people in your class who are going through the same things you are and who can help you. Get together with classmates whose skills and weaknesses are similar to yours and form study groups. Share tools, test each other, and talk about ideas with each other. This way of learning together can not only help you understand the subject better, but it can also help you make friends and feel like you belong in the medical school community.

Family and Friends: Your family and friends can always love, support, and encourage you, even if they don't fully understand how hard medical school is. Stay in touch with them, tell them about your events, both good and bad, and let them be your emotional anchor. It can help to know that you have strong support at home, even if they are not directly involved in medicine. This can give you a sense of security and comfort during hard times.

Mentors and advisors in medical school: Ask experienced faculty, doctors, or upperclassmen for help. They can give you useful information about the medical field, like how to do well on clinical rotations or how to apply for training. A lot of medical schools have programs that pair students with workers with more experience. Don't be afraid to talk to professors whose work interests you or talk to upperclassmen who seem friendly and ready to share their knowledge. Their advice can be very helpful as you go through medical school and deal with both classroom and professional issues.

Professionals in mental health: If you're having trouble with worry, anxiety, or other mental health issues, don't be afraid to get help from a therapist or counselor. A therapist can give you a safe place to talk about your problems, come up with ways to deal with them, and build your mental strength. They can give you tools and advice on how to deal with stress, keep a good work-life balance, and put your mental health first while you are in medical school.

Keeping in touch with people

Putting together a support system is one thing, but keeping it up and running takes work. Here are some ideas:

Set regular times: Don't let studying take over your whole life. It's important to spend time with family and friends, whether it's a weekly phone call or regular study breaks with coworkers. A well-balanced schedule with time for socializing and relaxing will help you avoid burnout and build better relationships with the people who help you.

Talk to your support network in an open and honest way. Share your experiences, both the good and the bad. Being honest with your loved ones builds trust and helps them understand what you're going through. Holding your feelings inside can make you feel alone and make it harder for the people you care about to help you in the ways you need them most.

Say "Thank You": Tell your friends, family, and teachers how much you appreciate their help. Tell them how grateful you are for their support and help. Taking the time to say thank you makes your relationships stronger and shows how important your support network is.

Also, be a friend who helps you. Remember that help works both ways. Also be there for your friends and teachers. Listen to them, celebrate their wins, and give them support when they're having a hard time. Strong ties that work both ways help build a sense of community and make the support network stronger for everyone.

In conclusion

A good support system will help you a lot as you go through medical school. Keeping in touch with friends, family, and mentors will help you build a network of support, encouragement, and well-being that will help you get through the tough times, enjoy the wins, and eventually reach your goal of becoming a great medical professional. Don't forget that you're not alone in this. Surround yourself with upbeat, helpful people who believe in you and what you can do. You'll be ready to handle the challenges of medical school and start a rewarding job in medicine if you have strong support around you.

CHAPTER 12

FINDING BALANCE

A Life Outside of Medicine

The draw of the white coat and the good cause of medicine can be too much to handle. Medical school gives you the skills you need for a successful job, but it's only the start of a journey that will last a lifetime. This chapter talks about how important it is to have a life outside of medicine, a good work-life balance, and to follow your interests outside of school.

Why hyperfocus is appealing and why it's dangerous

Focusing on your studies is important for doing well in school, but ignoring other parts of your life can cause burnout, less drive, and even health issues, both physical and mental. To find a balance between schoolwork and personal well-being, you don't have to get a perfect 50/50 split. Instead, you need to find a rhythm that lets you do well in both areas. **Here's why it's important to find balance:**

Fighting Burnout: Medical school is hard work with long hours, a lot of pressure, and what seems like an endless amount of knowledge to take in. Not spending time on your hobbies and interests can make you tired, cynical, and emotionally distant. Stress needs to be released, and doing things you enjoy will help you do that. Then you can go back to studying with more focus, energy, and a better attitude. Making plans for fun things to do isn't a sign of weakness; it's an investment in your long-term success.

Boosting Creativity and Problem-Solving: Taking a break from medicine and pursuing your interests can help you think of new ways to do things. Bringing different experiences and points of view to the table can help you solve problems better and change the way you care for patients in the future. As an example, a medical student who used to play music might approach a complicated medical case with a deeper understanding of rhythm and time, which could come in handy for tasks that need precise hand-eye coordination. In the same way, a student who loves writing might be great at making patient education tools that are clear and to the point.

Maintaining Physical and Mental Health: Doing well in school is important, but it shouldn't come at the cost of your physical and mental health. Several things can improve your health when you do things you enjoy. Getting some exercise, like playing a team sport, going for a jog by yourself, or taking a dance class, can really help you relax and feel better. Regular exercise is good for your heart, lowers your chance

of getting chronic diseases, and helps people who are depressed and anxious. Your general health can also be greatly improved by doing things that help you
relax and be more aware, like yoga, meditation, or spending time in nature.

Strengthening Relationships: For a good work-life balance, it's important to spend time building relationships with family and friends. A strong network of friends and family can help you deal with worry and give you hope when things are tough. Family and friends can give you a safe place to let off steam, celebrate wins, and just enjoy each other's company. Ignoring these relationships in order to focus only on schoolwork can make you feel alone and isolated, which can make your stress worse and hurt your grades.

Building a Life Besides Medicine

Being perfect isn't the point of finding balance; the point is to choose to fit activities you enjoy into your busy routine. Here are some ways to make your life more satisfying outside of medicine:

Find Your Passions Again: Think about the things you liked to do before you started medical school. What things made you happy and gave you a sense of accomplishment?

How did it feel to play the guitar? Did you read a lot? You might have helped at an animal shelter nearby. You should try to get these things back into your life, even if they have to be changed because of the time limits of medical school. Joining an online book club or practicing your guitar for a short time can get you excited about things again and give your mind a much-needed break.

Discover New Interests: Medical school doesn't mean you can't do other things. Now is the time to find and explore. You could join a book club, take a dance class, or help out a cause that you care about. Getting out of your comfort zone and trying new things can make your life better and help you find new interests. Through your charity work, you might find that you have a hidden talent for painting or that you become deeply interested in fighting for public health.

Schedule Time for Fun: Just like you schedule time to study and go to class, you should also schedule time for fun things. Give these things the same amount of value as your schoolwork. You should set aside certain times on your calendar to do things like sports, social events, or just reading a book. If you treat these events as important meetings, they won't get pushed aside by schoolwork.

Set Limits: Being able to say "no" is an important skill for keeping a good work-life balance. Although being dedicated is important, don't feel like you have to take on every extra task or activity that comes your way. Look at your work load and put your health first. You can focus on your main tasks and keep a steady pace if you say no to extra commitments.

Be a part of the journey: medical school is a stop on the way to becoming a doctor. Don't lose sight of the bigger picture: your love of medicine and the job you want to have in the future. When you find balance, you can go back to studying with new drive and a good attitude. Don't forget that taking care of yourself and pursuing your interests outside of medicine will make you a better, more well-rounded, and caring doctor in the long run.

In conclusion

Finding the right mix between schoolwork and personal well-being isn't about getting it exactly right; it's about finding a rhythm that works for you in both areas. Going to medical school is hard, but it doesn't have to be your whole life. You can create a satisfying life outside of medicine by pursuing your interests, planning time for fun things, and setting limits. Remember that a well-rounded person is a better person. They are better at learning, caring for others, and becoming a doctor. So go out there and do well in school, but don't forget to enjoy life outside of medicine.

General Tips for Readers

"Med Student to Medical Marvel: Habits of Highly Effective Learners"

This book provides you with the skills and tactics you need to convert your medical school experience from a stressful slog to one of empowerment and productive learning. Here are some basic suggestions to bear in mind as you begin on this thrilling journey:

Embrace the Challenge: Medical school is rigorous, but also extremely rewarding. Accept the challenge, knowing that the information and abilities you learn will help many people.

Find Your "Why": Remind yourself why you've chosen this route. Is it a lifetime love for medicine? Want to assist others? Hold onto your "why" throughout difficult times and let it drive your motivation.

Prioritize Self-Care: You cannot pour from an empty cup. Prioritize getting adequate sleep, eating nutritious meals, and doing things you like. Taking care of oneself improves your attention, memory, and general health.

Develop a Growth Mindset: Be confident in your abilities to learn and progress. Challenges provide opportunity to acquire new tactics and improve one's learning effectiveness.

Don't Be Afraid to Ask for Help: Nobody succeeds in medical school alone. Don't be afraid to ask instructors, classmates, or tutors for clarification or help.

Acknowledge and appreciate your achievements, no matter how large or small. Acing a test, understanding a challenging idea, or completing a clinical rotation are all accomplishments worth celebrating.

Find Your Learning Style: This book includes a number of learning methodologies. Experiment and figure out what works best for you.

Create a Support System: Surround yourself with positive and encouraging individuals, including classmates, mentors, family, and friends. Their encouragement will be vital along this journey.

Maintain Balance: While medical school is essential, it is not everything. Maintain interests, spend time with loved ones, and participate in things other than medical. A balanced lifestyle leads to a more rewarding medical profession.

Be Patient With Yourself: Learning requires time and effort. Don't get disheartened if you don't understand an idea instantly. You will succeed if you persevere and work consistently.

Remember, "Med Student to Medical Marvel" is your guide along your trip. Use the ideas on these pages, modify them to fit your learning style, and trust in your ability to become a highly successful student and, eventually, a talented and caring medical wonder.

www.ingramcontent.com/pod-product-compliance
Lightning Source LLC
Chambersburg PA
CBHW050236230526
45470CB00005B/1984